THE BUSY MAN'S
SKINCARE GUIDE

A SIMPLE SYSTEM TO GET BETTER SKIN IN 30 DAYS

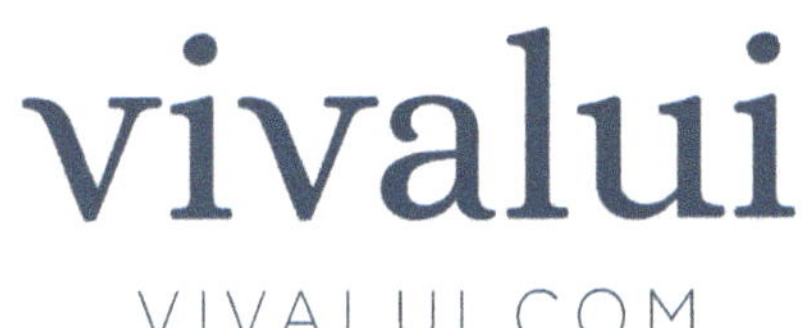

vivalui

VIVALUI.COM

TABLE OF CONTENT

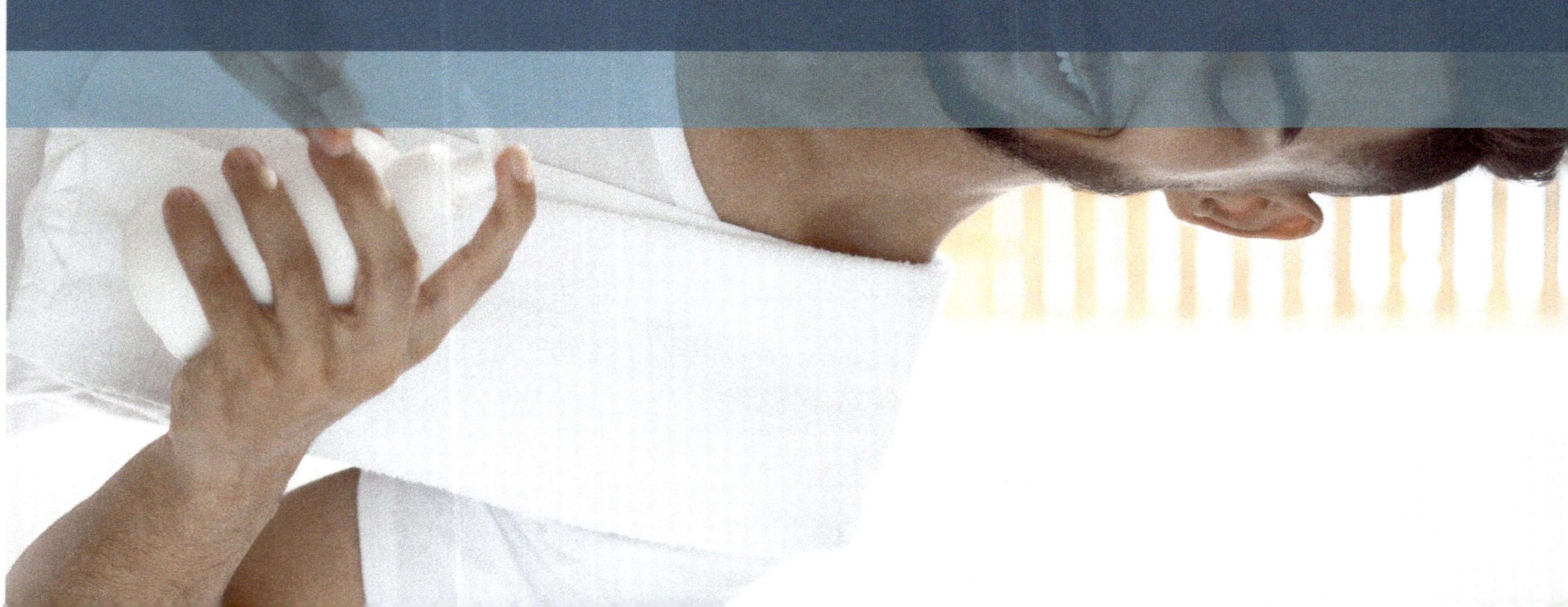

INTRODUCTION

INTRODUCTION

Once upon a time, men were expected not to care about their skin.

Being "rugged" was part of being a man, and taking care of how your skin looks was women's stuff.

Those times are (thankfully!) gone. Today, a man like you is expected to take care of his appearance, and take pride in it. To communicate, with how you look and dress, that you're in control. That you can be trusted to take care of things. That you're going places.

Let's be honest. It's hard to feel pride if your skin is not as it should be. You can have a great haircut, a good athletic body, clothes that fit you perfectly, and even a glorious beard. But if you have bad acne, heavy bags under your eyes, splotchy skin, or out-of-control wrinkles way too soon… that's what you will focus on every time you look in the mirror.

After all, your face is the first thing other people see, too.

Finally, a skincare guide for busy men.

We get it: you're busy. You have places to be, work to do.

You don't have time to sift through the thousands of low-quality articles about skincare on the internet (most of which are written for women's skin, anyway), or to even begin to make sense of the dozens of different product types and brands.

But still, you want the benefits of great skin. The confidence that comes from looking at the mirror and liking what you see. And the immense benefits that confidence can bring to your professional, romantic, and personal life.

And you know what? You deserve that. You deserve great skin.

That's why we built this guide.

Who is this guide for?

This guide is for any man who wants to have better skin.

Maybe you're a teenager or young man struggling with acne. Maybe you are a 30-something who wants to keep his skin looking young as long as possible. Maybe you're an older man looking to keep the wrinkles at bay.

It doesn't matter what you're struggling with, your skin tone, or your age. All that matters is that you want the beautiful, soft, glowing skin you deserve.

And if that's the case, keep reading.

Because this guide is for you.

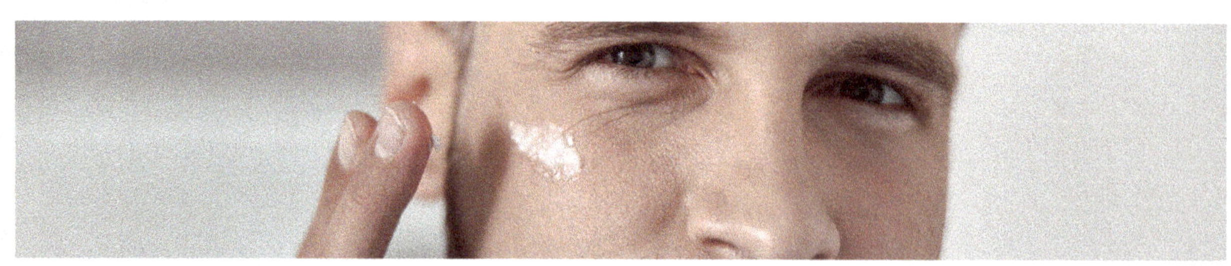

What can you expect from this guide?

In this guide, you will find a **complete system** you can use to improve the health and looks of your skin.

This system, unlike most of the online content on skincare, was designed *specifically for men* — because as we will see, men's skin can be very different from women's, and your skincare routine should take that into account. And it's based on the latest scientific evidence and on what works in the real world.

And since we know you're busy, we skipped all the theory and useless information. Instead, **we focused on action**. We laid out an entire plan for you to follow, with the specific changes you need to make to your daily routine to get the maximum benefit with the least effort.

The goal? To bring **real improvement** to your skin in just a few weeks.

Some important words before we start...

Proper skincare is a **holistic endeavor:** it's not just about what products you use in your routine, but also about what you eat, drink, and your overall life habits. In this guide, you will find specific tips to improve your lifestyle (and your skin).

In fact, your skin's health is tied to your overall health. And the good news is, as you apply these tips, you'll not just improve your skin: you'll get other benefits too!

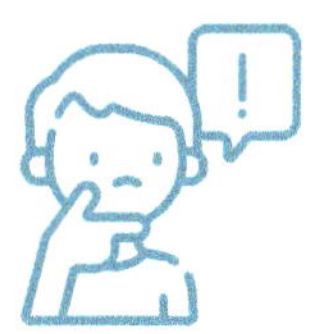

REMEMBER:

You don't have to be perfect to get the benefits! It's better to apply just a few of these tips than none at all. And it's better to follow them only when you can than never doing it at all.

So don't get discouraged if your current lifestyle makes some of the points in this guide impossible to follow. Feel free to pick and choose. Implement the "low hanging fruit" first.

We guarantee you'll see benefits in just a few weeks.

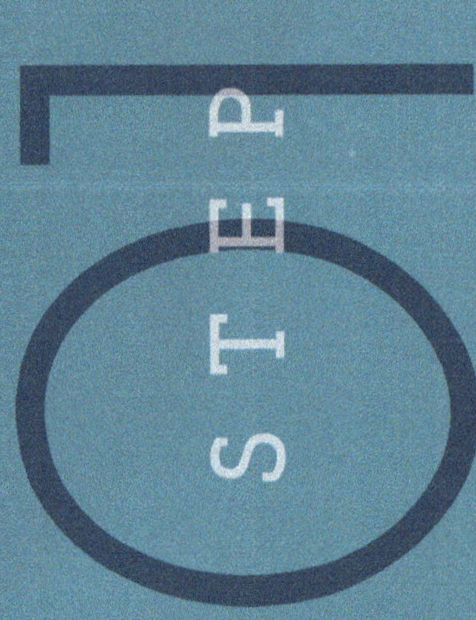

STEP
01
UNDERSTAND
YOUR SKIN

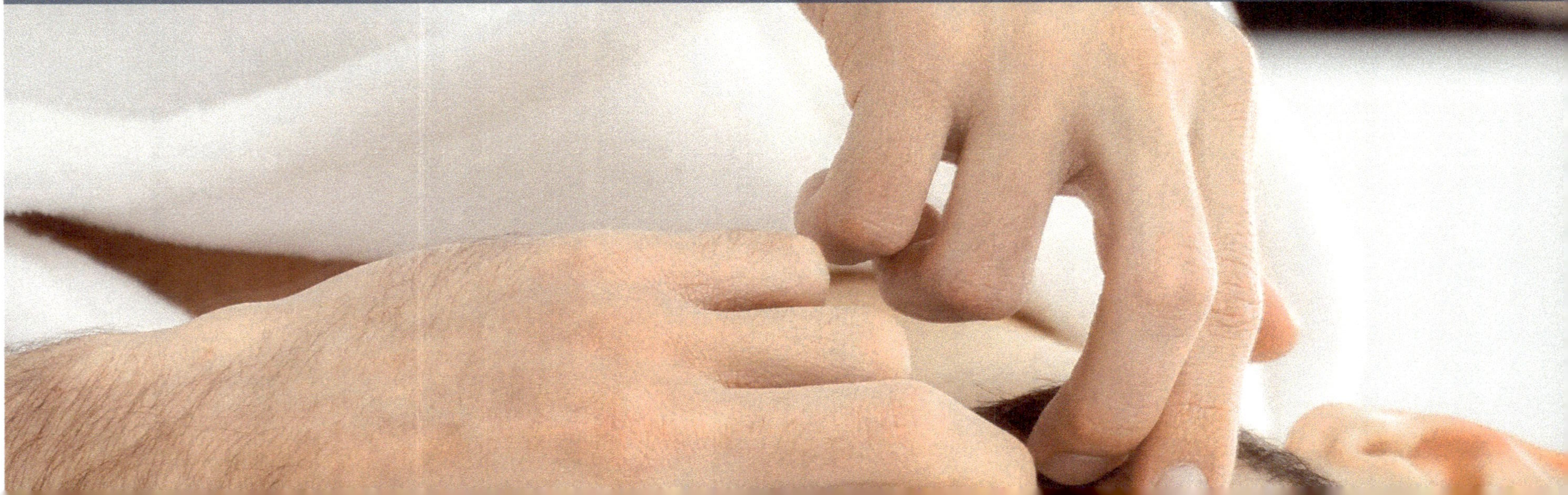

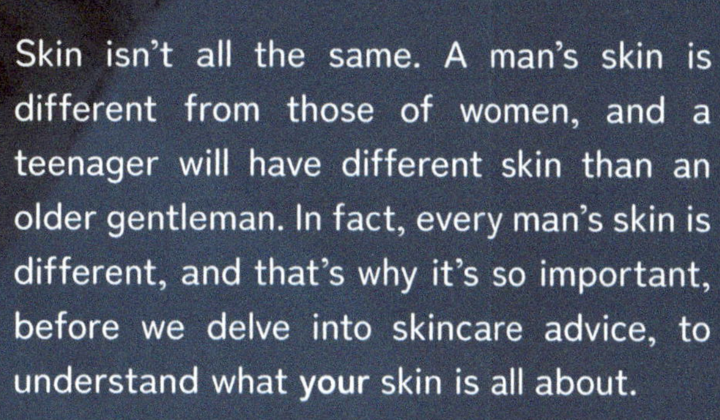

Skin isn't all the same. A man's skin is different from those of women, and a teenager will have different skin than an older gentleman. In fact, every man's skin is different, and that's why it's so important, before we delve into skincare advice, to understand what **your** skin is all about.

But don't worry! You're not in for a long, boring lesson.

Instead, we'll focus on practical, useful things. We'll try to understand how your skin is different from the skin of a woman (for whom most skincare content is written) and how to **find out what your type of skin is.**

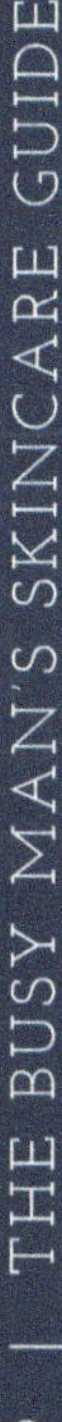

A Man's Skin Is Different

Most advice you can find on the web is geared towards women, and so are most skincare products. **But what about man's skin?** Can you use the same products? Does the same advice apply?

Yes and no. While it's still, of course, human skin, there are important differences between male and female skin — and when it comes to skincare, these differences matter.

Starting with puberty and adolescence, men and women go through very different hormonal changes. These different **hormones cause their skin to develop differently**. Thanks to testosterone and other androgenic (male-specific) hormones, your skin:

→ Is around **25% thicker** than a woman's, and has a tougher, rougher texture.

→ Has **more and bigger pores**, which produce more sebum (oil). This makes men more prone to severe acne.

→ Has **more collagen**, making it more flexible and making it age slower (although you wouldn't tell, since most men don't take care of their skin)

These differences matter for the formulation of skincare products, and that's why you should be careful to select products that are formulated specifically for men's skin.

Another important point to remember is that your skin is subject to **strong stressors during shaving.** Not just that, but traditionally most shaving creams were extremely aggressive on the skin and had high alcohol content, which dried it up — although that's changing in the last few years, as more and more men are taking an interest in skincare.

What's Your Skin Type?

When it comes to skincare, skin is divided into **five types,** each with its own issues and best practices.

It's important you **identify your skin type,** as your skincare routine and the products you use should be selected based on it.

Beware, however: **your skin type is not set in stone**. It depends not just on your genetics, but also on your conditions. Your age, stress, diet, lifestyle, and even the weather all factor in determining your skin type. Especially if you're a young man, you should be aware that your skin right now is probably not the same as it was at 15 or the one you'll have in 20 years.

Let's see what the five skin types are, so you can determine your own.

NORMAL SKIN

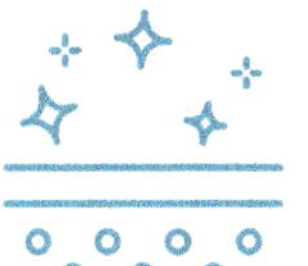

If your skin is not particularly oily or dry, and has an even tone without a lot of shine, cracks, or crispiness, then it's probably normal. In normal skin, pores are not obvious.

Men with normal skin should avoid products that break their skin's balance, making it too oily or too dry.

DRY SKIN

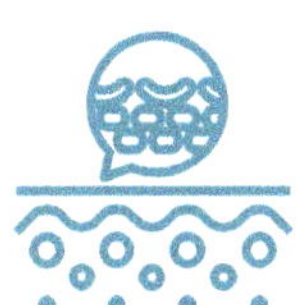

Dry skin has little oil production. If your pores are pretty much invisible, and your skin is dry with scaly patches and flaking, you probably have dry skin.

For men with dry skin, a good moisturizer is a must. Better if cream, as cream moisturizers have more oil and create a thicker lather on your skin.

OILY SKIN

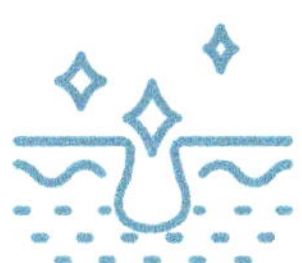

Oily skin has lots of oil. The skin appears shiny due to the oil, and is the type of skin that most tends to experience severe acne breakouts. If you suffer from diffuse acne and can easily feel the oil on your skin, you might have oily skin.

Men with oily skin need a good exfoliator in order to promptly remove dead cells that can block the pores and cause a breakout.

COMBINATION SKIN

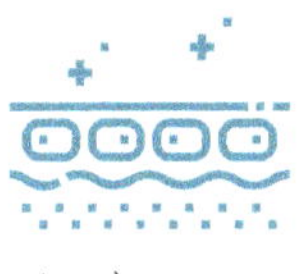

If your face has the characteristics of both dry and oily skin on different parts, it's probably combination skin. People with combination skin have dry sections while are oily in others. Often, the oily section is the T-zone (nose, forehead, chin).

This is the most common type of skin. A balanced skincare routine is the best way to take care of combination skin.

SENSITIVE SKIN

Sensitive skin can be dry, oily, or combination, but is also very prone to inflammation. If you often suffer from contact dermatitis or conditions like rosacea and allergic rashes, you have sensitive skin.

People with sensitive skin often shy away from skincare routines for fear of irritating their skin — but a balanced skincare routine is paramount to keep their skin protected against external agents that could irritate it! They should, however, avoid harsh chemical-based treatments. The more natural and delicate, the better.

STEP 02

GET HEALTHY SKIN HABITS

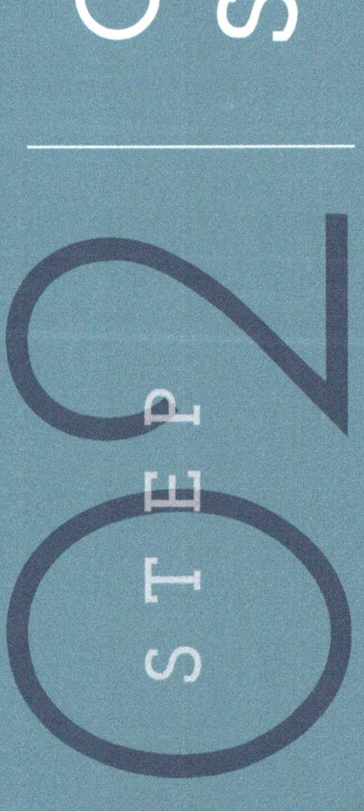

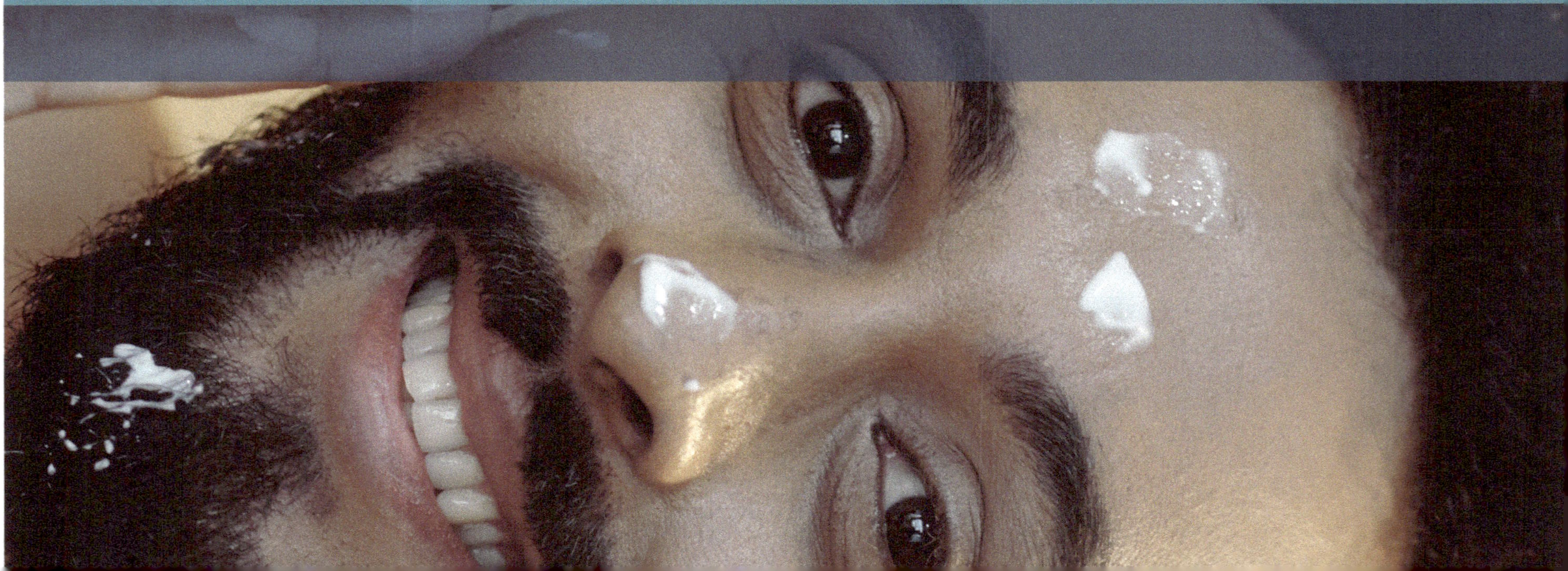

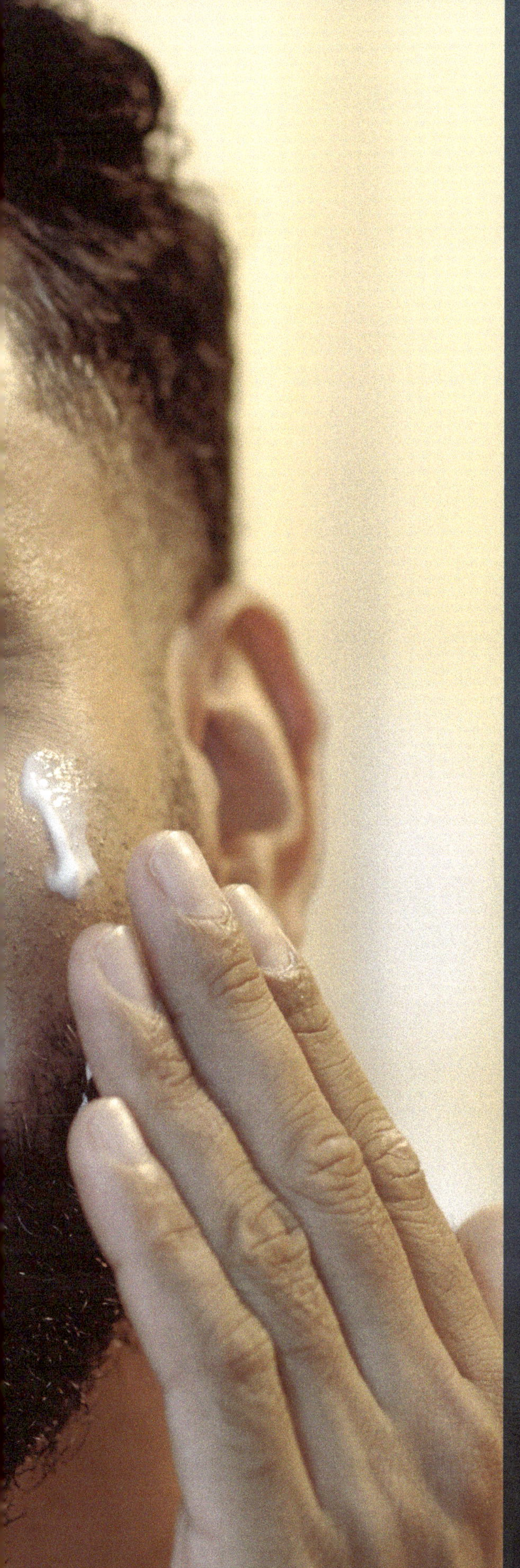

As we said in our introduction to this guide, **skin health is holistic:** it's not just about what you put on your face. Everything you do, from what you eat and drink to your sleeping habits has an effect on your skin.

But no reason to panic. It doesn't have to be complicated. In fact, taking care of just a handful of factors can get all the way from having bad skin to having beautiful, glowing skin.

In this section, you'll learn what **the most important things you can do for your skin are** — and how to do that in the simplest, most effortless way.

Avoid These Skin-Killer Foods…

Your skin is extremely sensitive to hormonal changes in your body, and what you eat has a large impact on your hormonal balance. So, it makes sense for what you eat to have an effect on your skin too.

Some foods are especially guilty of causing bad skin and promoting breakouts. Let's see what they are; in the next section, **we'll also see what to substitute them with.**

PROCESSED CARBS & HIGH SUGAR

Unsurprisingly, the #1 culprit is foods that are high in simple carbohydrates, specifically processed foods and foods with high sugar.

The problem is that these foods have a **high glycemic index.** That means they cause a spike in sugar blood, stimulating your body to produce insulin. Insulin, among other things, stimulates the oil glands in your skin, causing them to produce more sebum and therefore making your skin more prone to clogged pores and breakouts.

A good rule of thumb: **the more processed it is, the worse it is for your skin.**

- → Limit bread, pasta, candies, baked sweets, and processed food in general.
- → Go through your eating habits and evaluate what you can substitute for more natural foods.

EXTRA SALTY FOOD

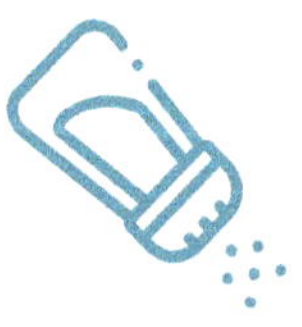

Food that is too rich in salts, while tasty, has a negative effect on your skin.

Salt causes dehydration and tenses the skin. The results are puffiness and bloating of your face, bulgy eyes, and dark circles. Research also shows too much salt is **connected to an increase in outbreaks.**

Of course, too much salt is not good for the rest of your body either.

- → Avoid extra salty snacks like potato chips, pretzels, and popcorn. Choose low salt alternatives where possible.
- → Use less salt in your own cooking, and be sure to rinse canned goods before consuming them (they're stored in a salty solution).

MILK & DAIRY

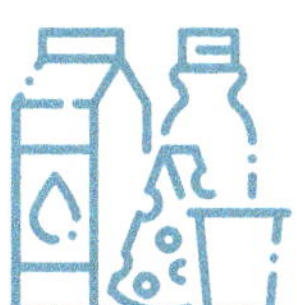

Milk and dairy products are rich in nutrients and hormones that impact your body and skin hormonal balance. They're associated with more clogged pores, and therefore to more acne breakouts, whiteheads, and blackheads.

One of the reasons is probably **prolactin**, a hormone found in milk that promotes the overgrowth of skin cells — making it more likely your pores will clog.

Avoid dairy products in your diet as much as possible.

Substitute milk with non-dairy alternatives, like soy milk or almond milk.

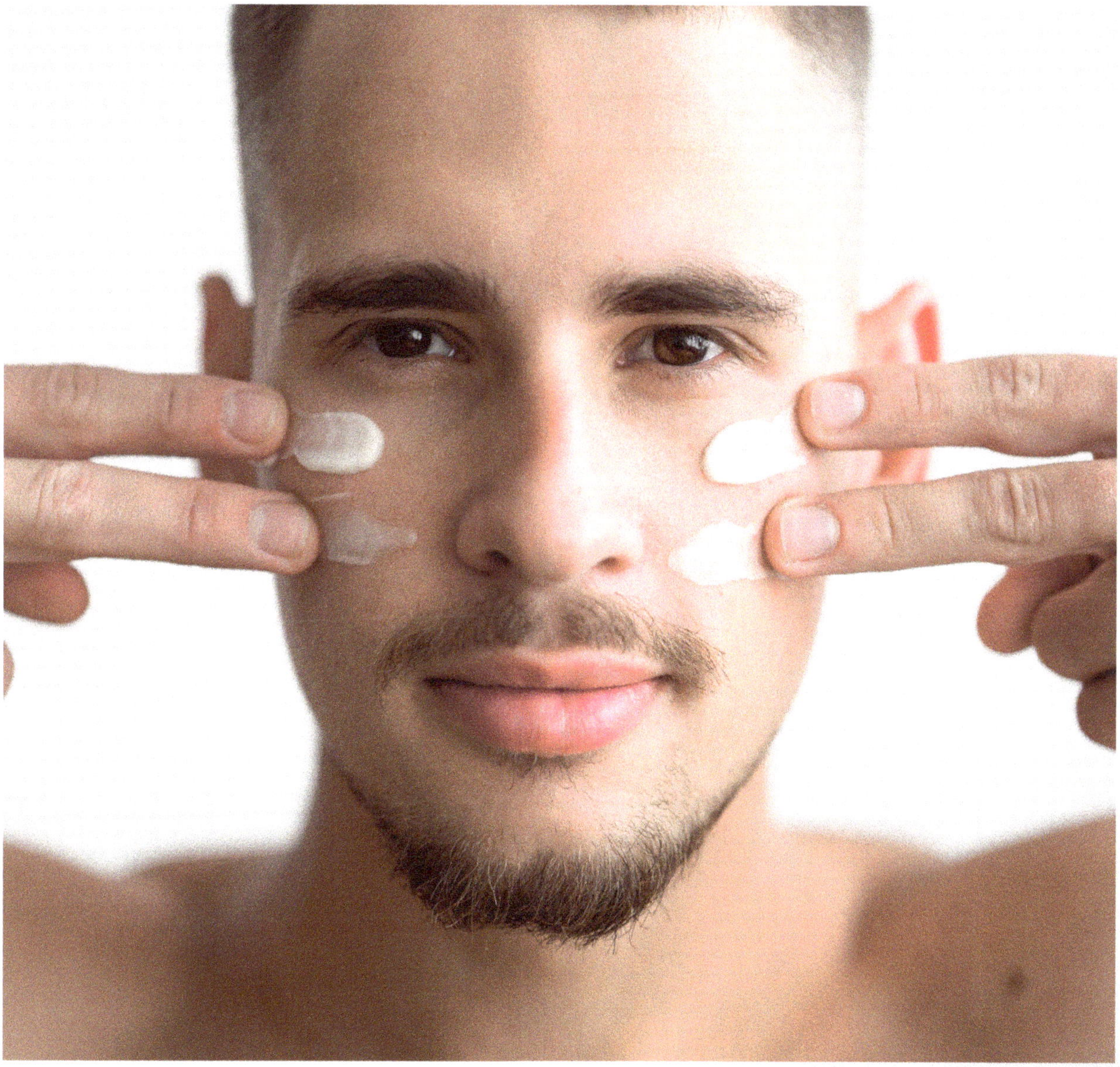

... Eat These Foods Instead!

The good news is that, while many foods in your diet might be making your skin worse, there's plenty of foods that can have **enormous benefits** for your skin (and overall health). And they're delicious, too!

Changing your eating habits can be hard. The key is to **make it a system**: don't just make a point to avoid bad foods in the future, but come up with specific substitutions. For example, if you usually have a candy bar snack at work, think about what you could bring instead. Implement that change into your life immediately.

Here are a few skin-enhancing foods you can introduce into your routine.

FOODS RICH IN HEALTHY FATS

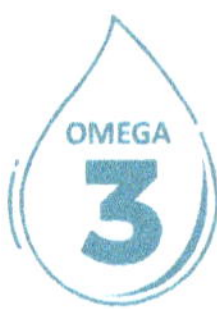

Many fatty acids are critical to our body's and skin's health, but our body cannot produce them directly. That's why we need to add them to our diet.

When it comes to the skin, these acids have an important role in **preventing inflammation** and keeping the skin hydrated and free of wrinkles. They also have been shown to protect against skin cancer and reduce acne.

The most famous of these acids are the **Omega 3s**, found in fatty fish like salmon and tuna, in walnuts and soybeans, and in seeds like flaxseed and chia seeds. Another important one is **oleic acid,** found in olive oil, avocados, almonds, and some nuts like macadamia nuts.

- → Look up recipes and substitute some of your meals with fatty fish.
- → Cook using olive oil to get oleic acid in your diet.
- → Substitute processed carbs snacks with nuts, walnuts, almonds, and seeds.

DARK CHOCOLATE

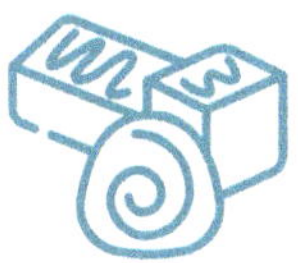 Did not expect to find chocolate here, did you? After all, it's folk wisdom that chocolate causes breakouts.

That may be true, but it's mostly due to the sugar and additives you find in most chocolate bars. Luckily, you don't have to swear off chocolate altogether!

Dark, sugar-free chocolate is rich in **flavonoids,** natural antioxidants that help prevent aging and sun damage, while also promoting a healthy glow of your skin. So you can use dark chocolate as a treat to satisfy your sweet tooth.

Introduce dark chocolate as a treat at the end of your meals or as a snack instead of processed candy bars.

GREEN AND ORANGE-YELLOW VEGETABLES

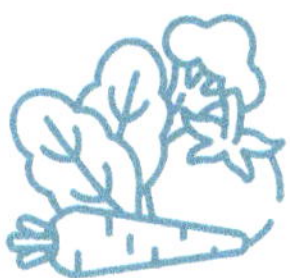 Unsurprisingly, vegetables (including fruit) are great for your skin — and of course, for your overall health too.

In fact, both **leafy greens and orange-yellow vegetables** contain a host of nutrients that are *critical* to your skin. Among these, **carotenoids** like lutein and lycopene are antioxidants that help protect your skin from the sun and other oxidative damage.

So make sure your fridge is always well stocked!

→ Introduce abundant vegetables into your diet.
→ Use vegetables like carrots and grapefruit as tasty alternatives to salty snacks.

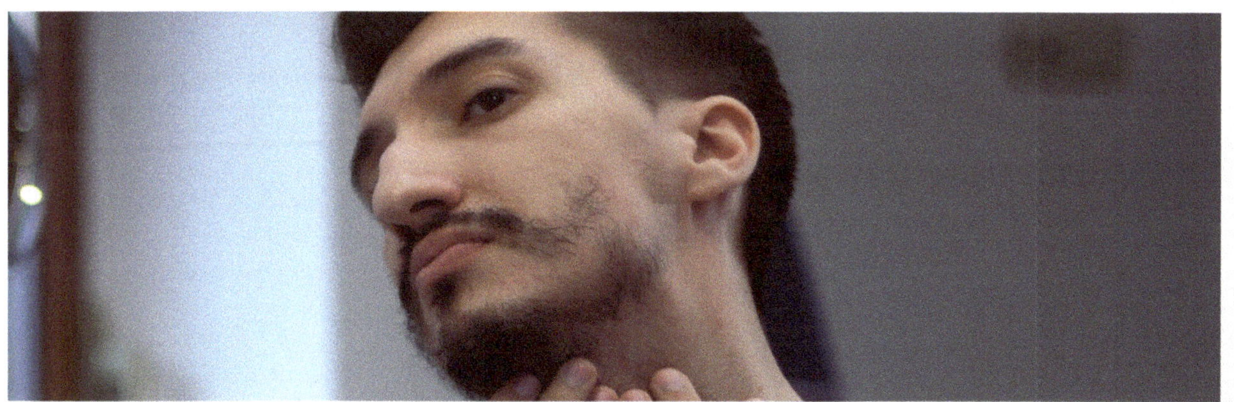

Limit These Drinks...

Just like food, what you drink influences your health. After all, **drinks have nutrients and hormones in them**, just like food, and they can be processed just as much.

While it's harder to substitute some beverages than it is to substitute foods, if you care about your skin it's worth thinking about how you can strategically change your drinking habits. In the sections below, we added some tips that should make it easier.

Here are three drinks that have a bad effect on your skin.

ALCOHOL

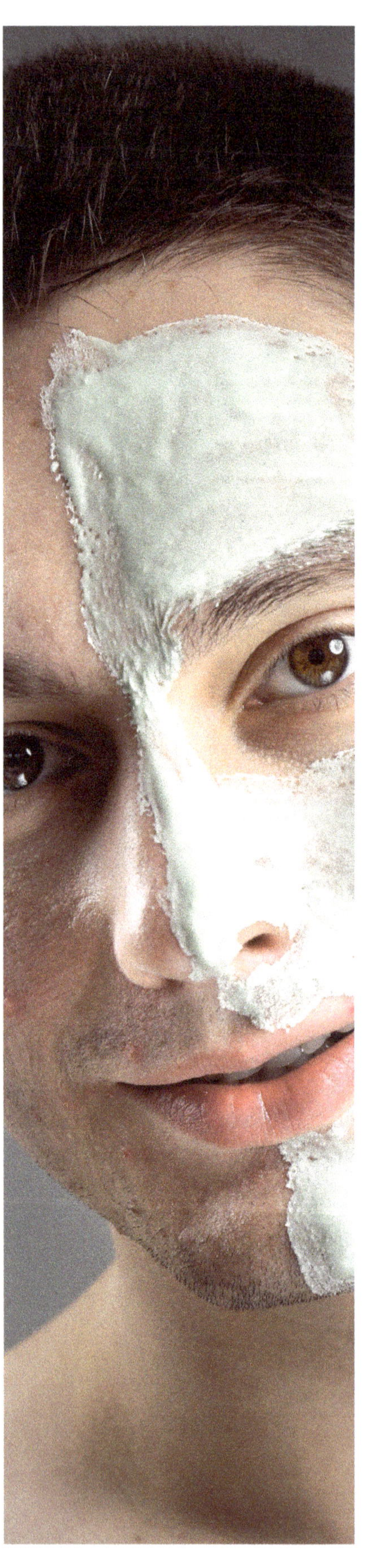

Too much alcohol is of course not good for your body, and your skin is no exception.

It **dehydrates the skin**, making it more vulnerable to bacteria and breakouts. Not only that, but alcohol depletes the body of important vitamins and minerals.

In particular, it depletes the body's supply of **vitamin A**, which is important for skin renewal and repair. Studies show alcohol consumption is associated with skin conditions such as eczema, acne, psoriasis, and rosacea.

Of course, as long as you don't abuse it, it's fine to have a drink or two!

→ Limit alcohol to two drinks.

→ Prefer beer or wine to harder drinks with higher alcohol content.

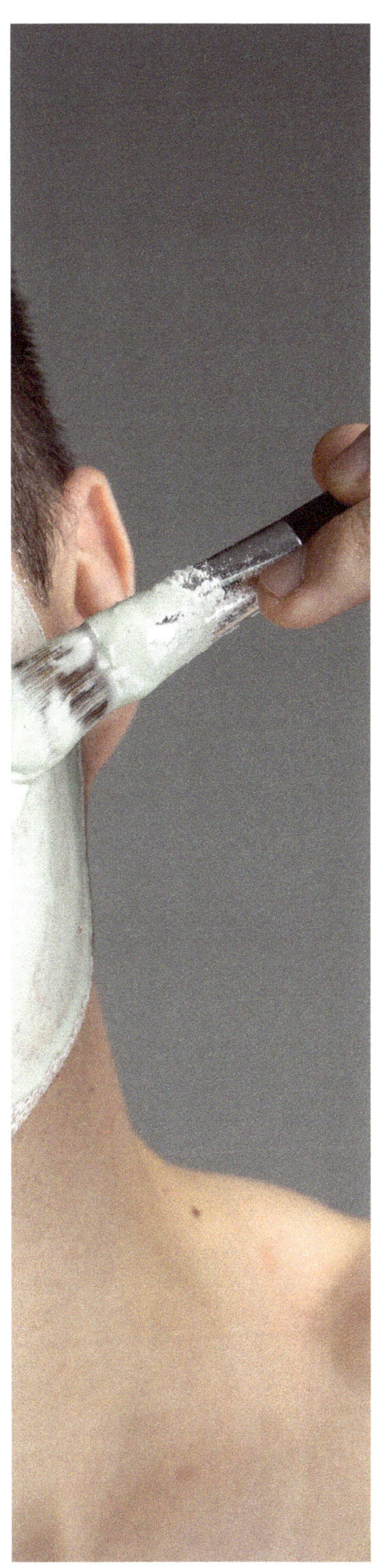

COFFEE

Unfortunately, coffee isn't that good for your skin, either.

Not only is it a diuretic, promoting dehydration, but most of all it causes a **spike in cortisol**, also called the stress hormone. Do you know how they say stress makes you look older? It's true. Cortisol causes your skin to age faster, makes it thinner, and leads to wrinkles.

Of course, you don't have to cut out coffee entirely. But it's worth thinking about avoiding abusing it.

→ Limit the coffee you drink during your day. Substitute some cups with decaf coffee or tea.

SUGARY DRINKS

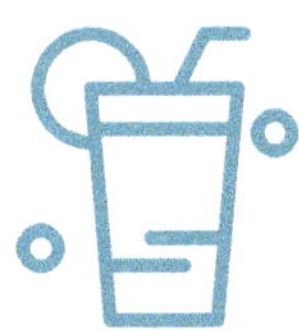

This should not come as a surprise. Sodas and processed juices are extremely **rich in sugar**, and the same argument we made for sugar-rich foods is just as true for them.

To make things a bit better, in the last few years the market has become richer with much healthier choices, which we suggest you prefer every time you can.

→ Prefer diet sodas to the traditional sugar-rich version of your favorite beverages.

→ Drink freshly squeezed fruit juice instead, or even flavored water.

.. AND GET MORE WATER

Drinking enough water is obviously important. But did you know that dehydration is one of the worst things you can do for your skin?

If your body doesn't get enough water, your skin won't have the reservoir of water it needs to hydrate properly. That results in itchy, inflammation-prone skin, with dark circles under our eyes and more fine lines and wrinkles.

Now, here's something you probably don't know: **if you drink when you're thirsty, you are already dehydrated!**

In fact, if you hydrate correctly, you should never feel "thirsty". Most people are actually walking around constantly dehydrated, and their skin suffers from it.

Recommendations on how much water to drink vary depending on the source, and of course, people of different sizes need different amounts of water. But it's easy to make sure you're not dehydrated without overdoing it.

Here's a **simple system** to make sure you get enough water. Make sure you drink a glass or cup of water at these daily "milestones":

- → As soon as you wake up
- → After your breakfast
- → Before lunch
- → Before your mid-afternoon snack
- → Before dinner
- → Before going to sleep

Since these cups of water are just before meals, it's easy and convenient. All you need to do is remember to drink before starting your meal, and just after/before getting into bed.

Of course, if you work a physical job or practice sports, you need to add the necessary hydration to this plan. But just by following this plan, you'll make sure you are regularly getting your body the water it needs.

Please notice that beverages like coffee, tea, and sodas are not included in this plan. Don't make the mistake of considering your morning coffee as your wake-up cup of water!

Try These Supplements

Nutritional supplements are a great way to make sure your body is getting all the nutrients it needs to keep your skin healthy and beautiful.

While you can technically get all these nutrients from your diet, **most people don't get nearly enough.** So if you care about your skin, it's worth thinking about a stack of supplements that gets your skin where it should be.

Modern supplements are safe and effective, and the nutrients we suggest below can be found in most multivitamin compounds. Just make sure you don't take more than the indicated dose, and you'll be fine. It's easy to **make a habit out of taking your supplements** with a meal (usually, lunch), and the benefits for your skin can be enormous.

Without further ado, let's see what the most important nutrients for your skin are!

ZINC

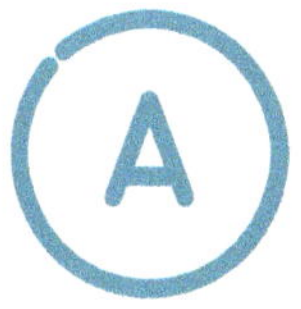

Zinc is a mineral that is involved in hundreds of important processes in our body, from regulation to wound healing.

When it comes to your skin, zinc helps in multiple ways: it reduces inflammation and helps regulate the production of sebum. It also has a role in regulating cell reproduction and death, reducing the excessive buildup of dead skin cells.

Research shows that there is a **correlation between zinc deficiency and severe acne.** Not just that, but there is evidence that zinc supplementation helps reduce acne breakouts and their severity.

VITAMIN A

Vitamin A is an important vitamin for your skin's health, and it comes in two types: **retinoids** and **carotenoids**. Both are present in many of the foods recommended in this guide, but it's important to make sure you're getting enough.

Vitamin A has an important role in regulating the skin's metabolic cycle, helping to keep the balance of oil production and dead skin cells healthy.

There is evidence that vitamin A helps reduce acne, stimulates collagen production, and reduces wrinkles. In general, it's essential to your skin.

In fact, **retinol creams,** which are skin products used to reduce wrinkles and signs of aging, are simply vitamin A in topical form.

Just a word of warning regarding supplements: unlike most nutrients, too much vitamin A can be toxic for your organs. This is not something you should be worried about, as long as you follow the recommended dosages.

VITAMIN E AND C

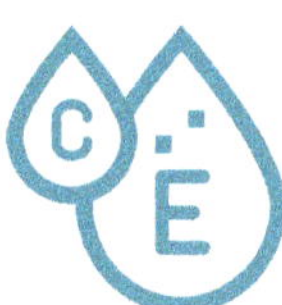

Vitamin E and C are powerful natural antioxidants, and studies show that their interaction is particularly important for their function.

Vitamin E has **powerful anti-aging effects on the skin**, protecting against signs of aging and soothing the skin. Scientific evidence shows Vitamin C has a boosting effect on Vitamin E's function, while Vitamin E itself acts as a stabilizer for Vitamin C.

Bottom line: make sure you're getting enough of both of them to keep your skin fresh and younger-looking.

VITAMIN B COMPLEX

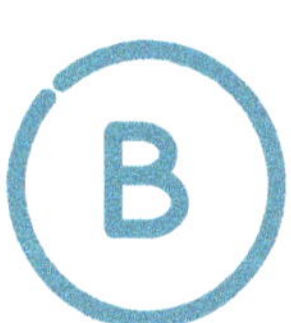

Vitamin B is a generic name for a **group of essential vitamins**, which includes riboflavin, thiamine, niacin, folate, inositol, pantothenate, choline, and biotin.

The vitamins in the B complex have fundamentally important roles to play in the healing and regenerating processes of the body, including the skin.

In fact, a deficiency in these vitamins can cause a series of **skin symptoms**: acne, rashes, flaky skin, and wrinkles. It also makes your skin more vulnerable to sunlight and easily irritable by external agents, including skincare products.

Sun, Sleep, And Soap

There are three critical factors for your skin's health that men are constantly ignoring. And your skin suffers for it.

Thankfully, they're easy to fix. So let's get right to it and find out how to make sure your habits are on point when it comes to sun, sleep, and soap!

WASH YOUR FACE THE RIGHT WAY

How to wash your face sounds obvious, right?

In fact, most men are hurting their skin by washing their face too much with aggressive soaps. Unlike what you might think, random bar soaps or even worse hand soaps should **never** touch your face.

Why? Bar soaps are aggressive and remove too much of the natural oils that protect your skin, causing your glands to overproduce oil to compensate. They also have an alkaline pH, throwing off the chemical balance of your skin and causing overgrowth of bacteria associated with breakouts.

→ Use a facial cleanser during your skincare routine, and avoid soaps during your day (just water is fine to refresh if you're not outright dirty).

→ Wash your face with lukewarm water, not too cold and not too hot.

→ To dry, pat your face with a towel instead of rubbing it.

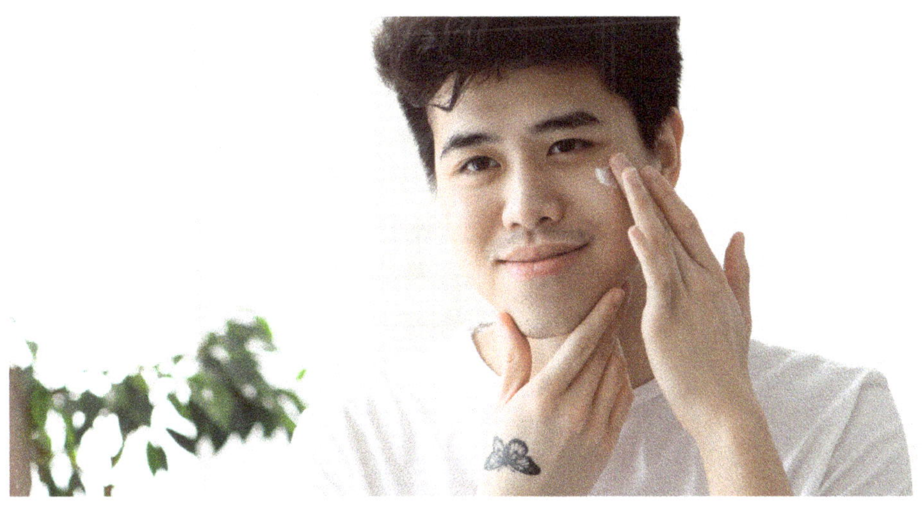

MIND THE SUN

Because they have more collagen, a man's skin ages much slower than a woman's. And yet, you can rarely see that on men's faces. Why's that?

The answer is that most men completely neglect sunscreen. They might use it on a beach day. But the truth is that solar radiation is the #1 factor in skin aging, and **sunscreen should be used every day**, even if you have darker skin.

Too much exposure can cause your skin to age prematurely, it can cause dark spots to appear (hyperpigmentation), and of course is a factor in skin cancer.

The American Academy of Dermatology recommends using a broad-spectrum sunscreen (which offers protection to UVA and UVB radiation) of 30 SPF at least, every day.

→ Apply proper sunscreen every day, at least 15 minutes before going out to give it time to affect your skin.

→ Choose a broad-spectrum sunscreen with 30 SPF protection.

PRIORITIZE YOUR SLEEP

You might not think your sleep matters to your skin health, but it's critical.

As you sleep, **your body heals and repairs its tissues**, and skin is no exception: during your sleep your skin renews, reducing inflammation and healing faster from breakouts and lesions. Bad sleep breaks this process, creating a more unbalanced skin that's more prone to getting inflamed.

→ Help your skin heal by making sure it's clean before sleeping with a good evening skincare routine.

→ Make sure you get 8 hours of sleep every night and try to keep your sleep time consistent to give your body rhythm.

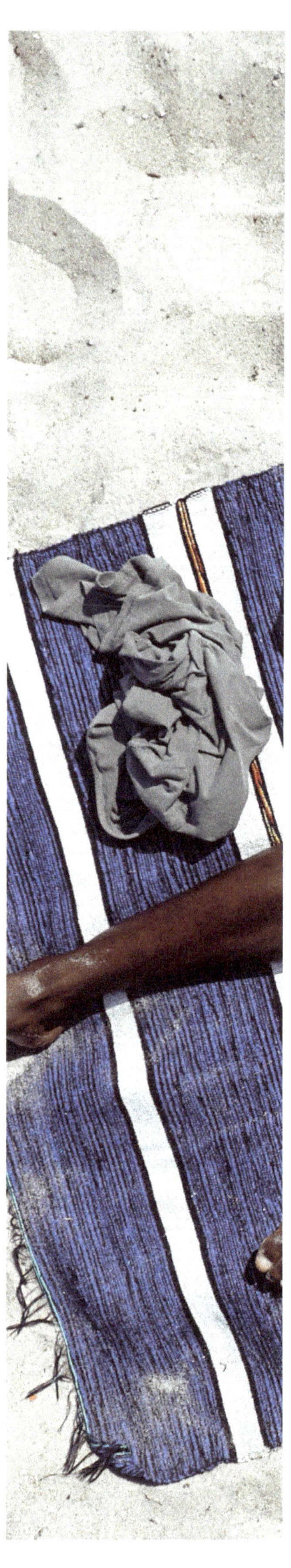

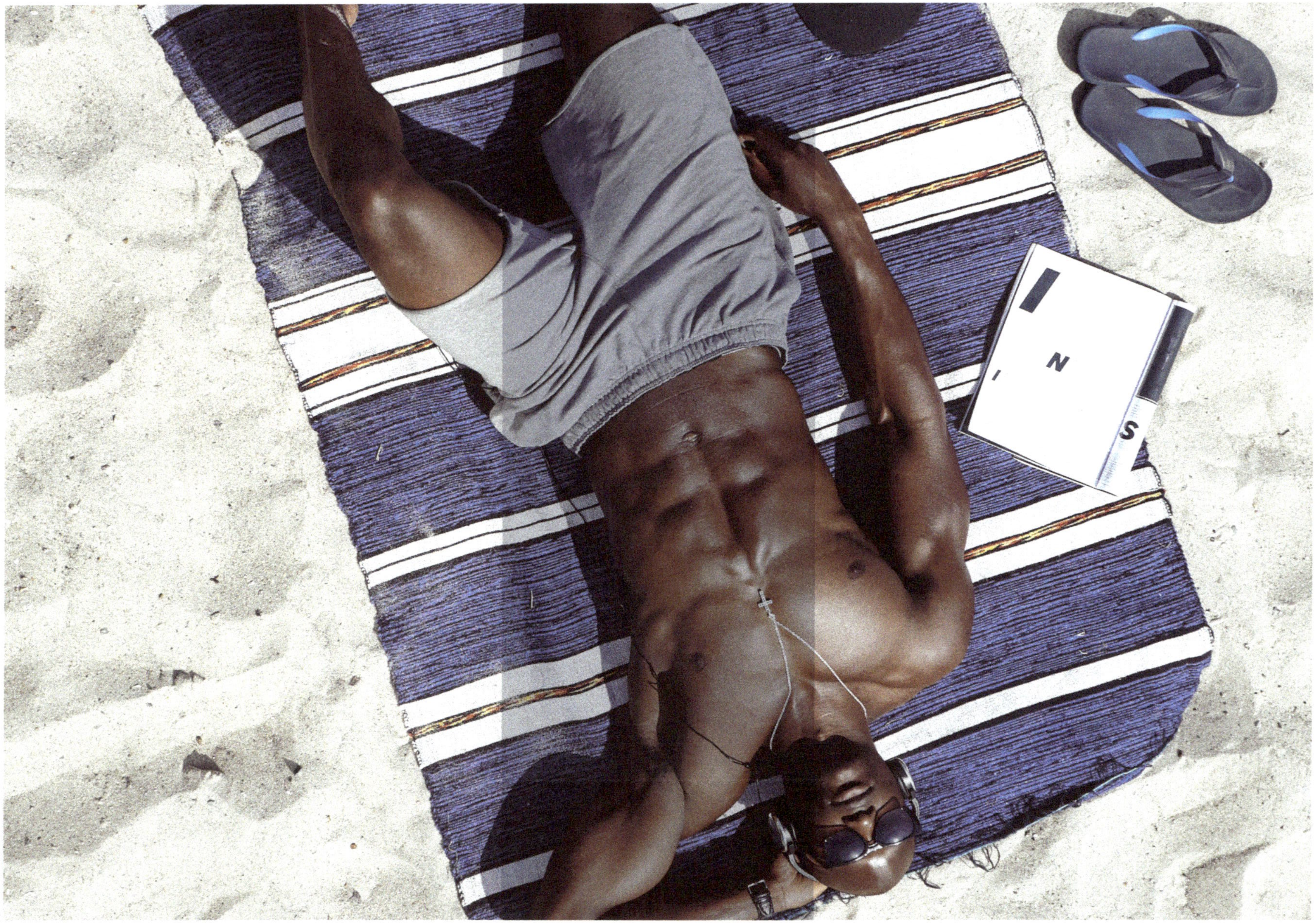

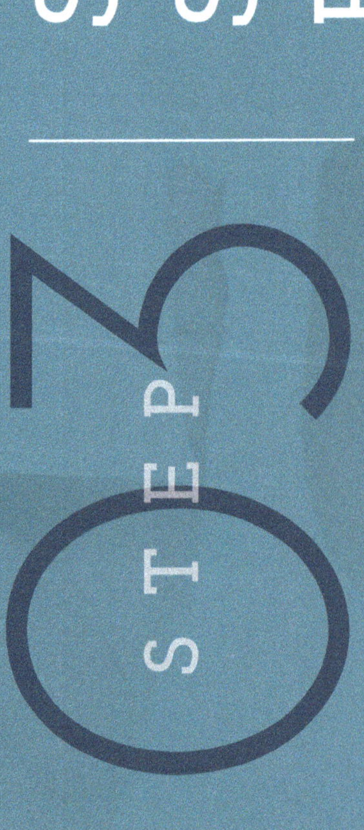

SET UP YOUR SKINCARE ROUTINE

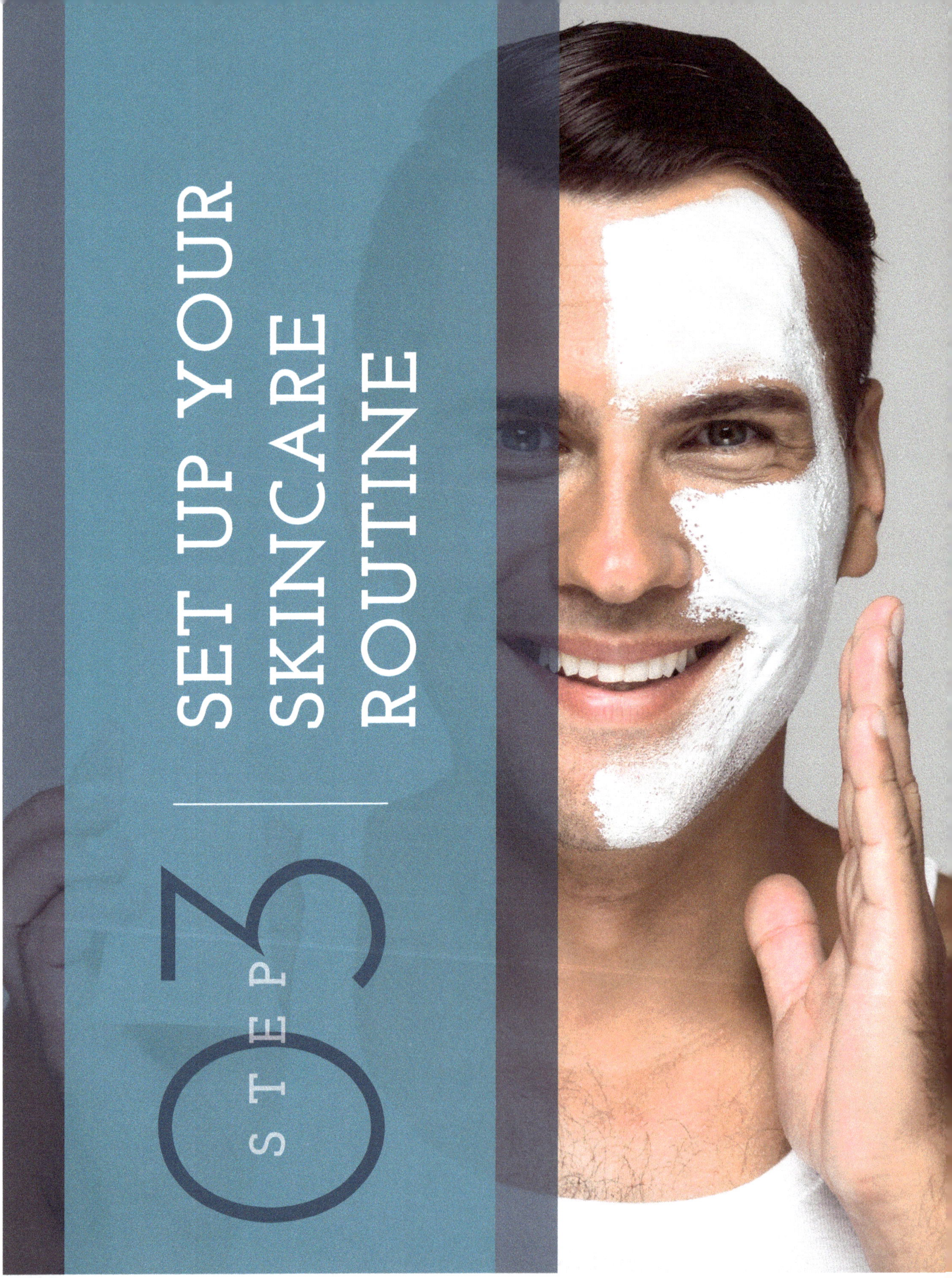

STEP

03

If you are like most men, you know little or nothing about skincare products and how to use them. In this last section of the guides, you'll learn all you need to know.

First, we'll go through the main types of products, and briefly explain what they do.

Then, we will share with you the **two skincare routines** we've prepared for you: a dead-simple one, great for beginners looking to get their feet wet with skincare; the other, more advanced, for those who want to go all the way.

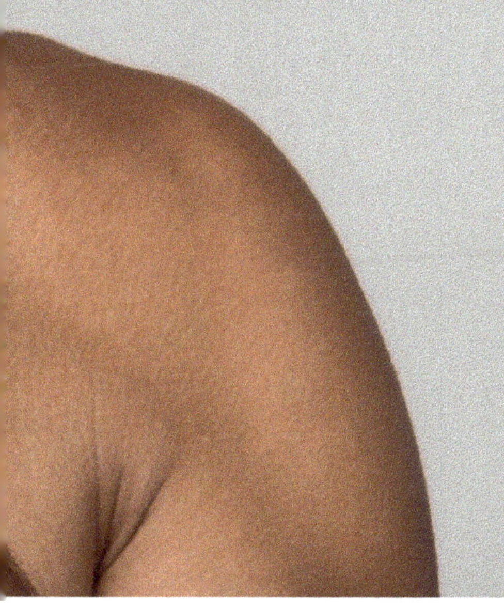

The Simple Skin Products Overview

For most men, the world of skin products is a mystery. Unlike women, most men haven't learned about them until later in life — and since most content and products are geared towards women, it's hard to understand what each product does and what they need.

No worries. **We're here to help.** In this section, we'll briefly go through the most important skincare products and explore what they do and what they're for.

Let's get started.

CLEANSERS

Cleansers are products meant to clear your face from oil, dead skin cells, dirt, and other external agents. They keep your pores clean, helping you keep breakouts at bay. Good cleansers respect your skin's natural pH, limiting dryness and irritation.

Cleansers come in many forms: gel cleansers are more indicated for oily skin types, while cream cleansers leave more oil on your face and are better for dry skin.

As we said earlier in this guide, you should not use standard soaps for your face — they're too aggressive. Cleansers are what you should use instead.

TONERS

Facial toners are products that refresh your skin. In short, what they do is hydrate your skin, thoroughly clean your pores, and remove excess oil, dead skin cells, and dirt from deep inside them.

A good toner is a game-changer if you suffer from breakouts and acne.

It's important to make sure the toner you choose is a good fit for your skin type. Most good toners come with specific instructions.

MOISTURIZERS

Moisturizers keep your skin hydrated by creating an isolating layer that keeps your skin's moisture inside. They also contain nutrients that nourish your skin.

Of course, dry skin types need moisturizers the most, but even if you have oily skin you should still use a (mild) moisturizer.

Many men hate the feeling of moisturizer on their faces. If you feel moisturizers are too heavy on your face, choose lotions and gel moisturizers instead of creams, as they are lighter.

EXFOLIATORS

Exfoliators are products that scrub your face from dead skin cells, helping you keep your pores clean and making your skin feel softer and smoother.

It's important to choose a gentle exfoliator, especially if your skin is sensitive because aggressive exfoliators can irritate your skin.

Exfoliating is not something you should do every day, but men should do it more often than women. Depending on the need, you can exfoliate twice or even three times a week.

MASKS

Masks are products that complement your skincare by sealing up your skin and delivering concentrated additives and nutrients. Often, masks are indicated for specific skin types and skin issues.

There are different kinds of masks, depending on what is used to seal the skin. For beginners, we recommend clay masks. These masks use clay and mud to clean deep into your pores.

You should always make sure your skin is clean and dry before applying a mask.

EYE CREAMS

Eye creams deliver concentrated nutrients to the skin around the eyes.

The skin around the eyes is thinner and more delicate than the rest of the skin on your face, and it has fewer oil glands, making it more prone to being dry. It's also more tense, due to the constant movement of the eyes.

Eye creams are a powerful ally against dark circles, bulgy eye bags, fine lines, and wrinkles, and we recommend them especially to gentlemen who are beginning to see signs of aging around the eyes.

SERUMS

Serums are concentrated formulations that deliver a high dose of nutrients to your skin to deal with specific issues, typically aging and skin damage.

They are made to be absorbed quickly, and contain ingredients like antioxidants and collagen, helping your skin recover from damage and stay young for longer.

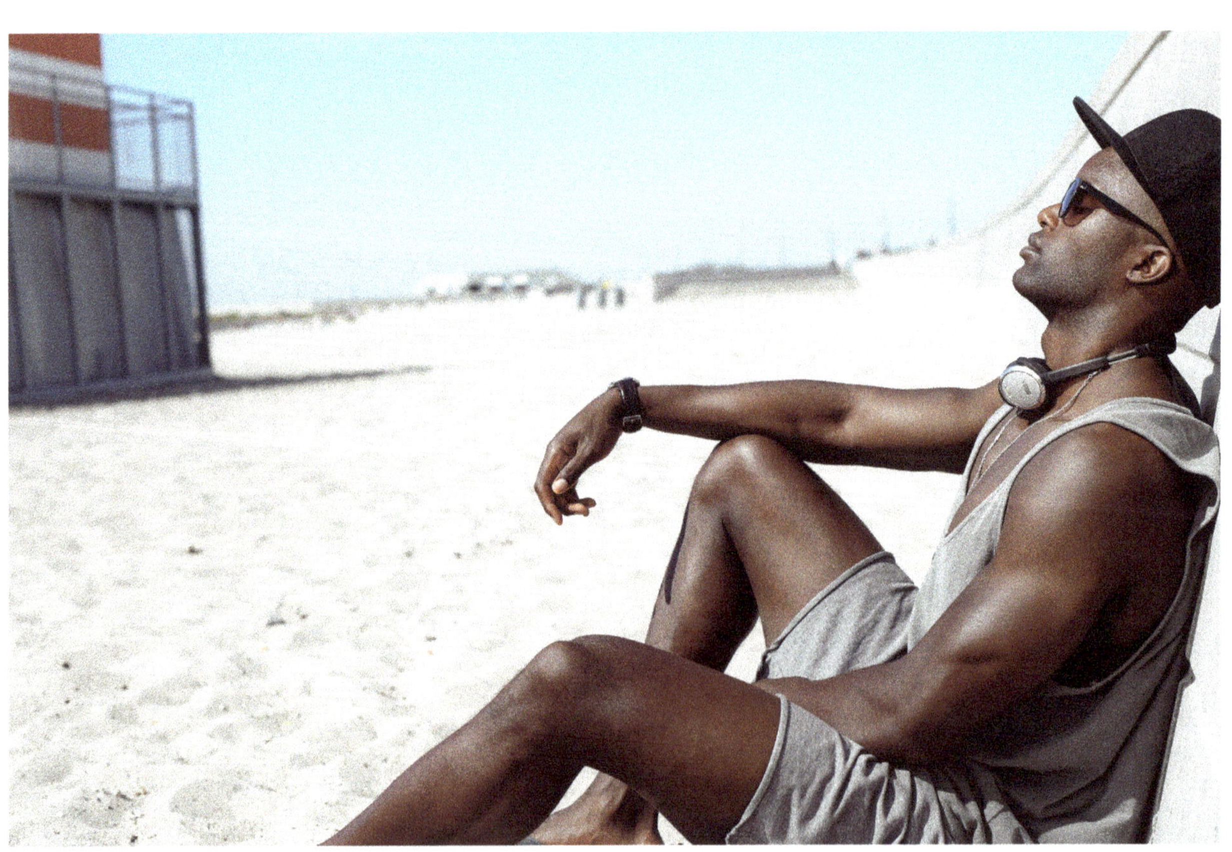

The Dead-Simple Skincare Routine

If you are a skincare beginner, or you're so busy you don't want to spend more than a few minutes dealing with it, this simple **3-step routine** is for you.

Including only the most important elements, it will give you the most bang for your buck and take almost no time. We also included a quick guide on each step, so you know exactly what to do!

This routine is meant to be repeated twice a day, in the morning and before you go to bed at night.

CLEANSER

As we said before in the guide, a cleanser is what you should use to keep your face clean instead of aggressive soaps.

→ Choose a cleanser that is specific to your skin type.

→ Splash warmish water on your face, and apply the cleanser clockwise. Rinse thoroughly and dry your face with a towel (pat, don't rub!)

→ If you are dealing with clogged pores and acne, consider adding an **acne toner** after your cleanser. Oily skin types can also benefit from using a **salicylic acid solution** to clean the excess oil from the face.

MOISTURIZER

A good moisturizer is a must, no matter your skin type. Most moisturizers will not just help keep your skin hydrated but also contain nutrients and ingredients to improve your skin's overall health.

→ Apply the moisturizer with your fingers, rubbing it in **circular motions** until you feel it's well absorbed.

→ If you have dry skin, choose a stronger moisturizer. If your skin is oily, choose a lighter product. As a rule, cream moisturizers tend to be stronger than gels.

SUNSCREEN

Sunscreen is a must to protect your skin from sun damage during the day and keep it young for longer. As we already mentioned in the relevant section:

→ Apply the sunscreen 15 minutes before going out to give it time to affect your skin.

→ Choose a broad-spectrum sunscreen (effective against UVA and UVB rays) with at least 30 SPF protection.

→ Of course, you don't need to apply sunscreen during your evening routine!

→ And that's it! Welcome to the wonderful world of skincare.

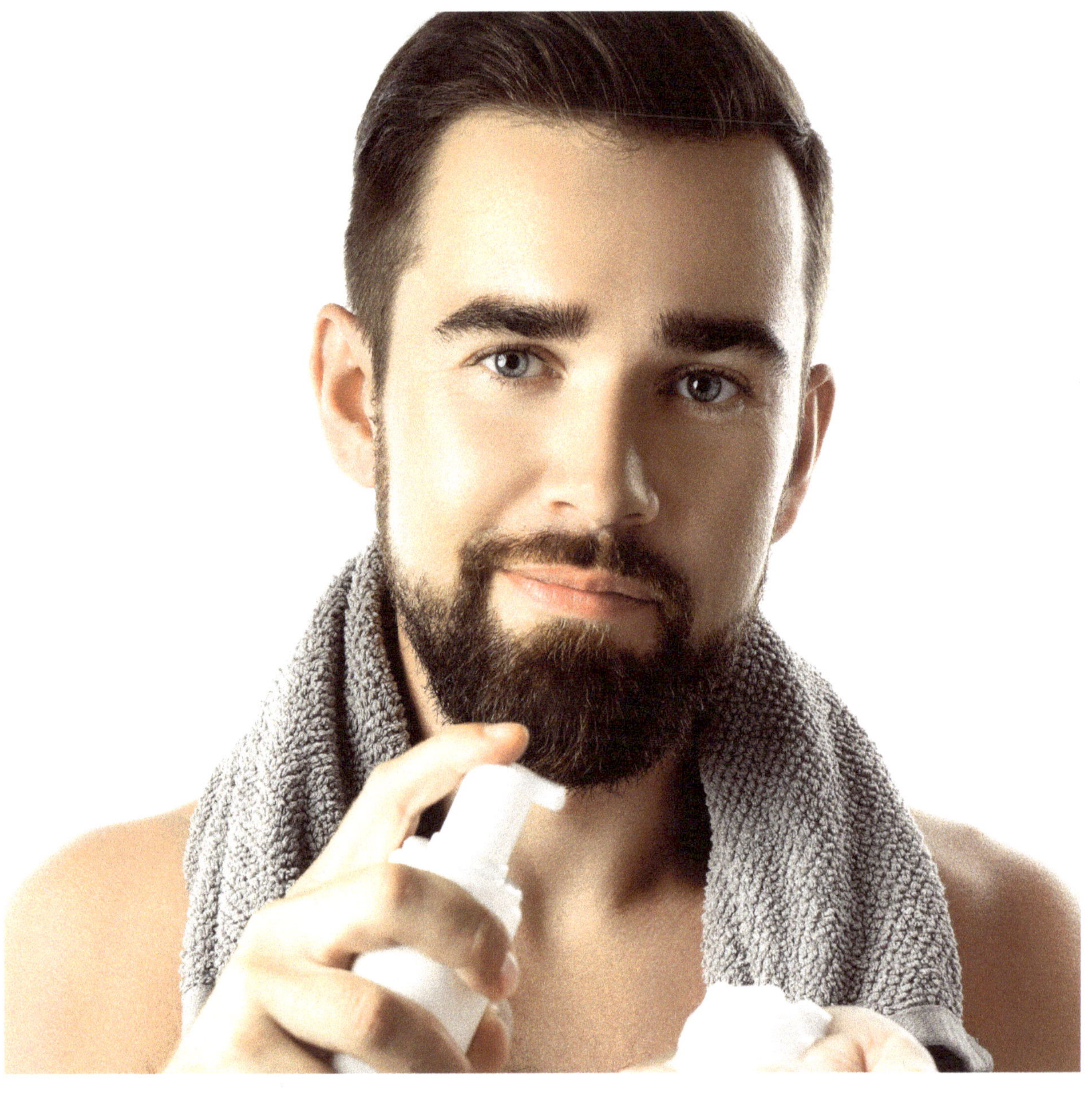

Advanced Skincare Routine

The simple skincare routine we just presented works great for beginners and people who are not experiencing serious skin issues. But what if you want to add something to it? What's the correct order?

In this section, we'll present you with the **correct sequence** to follow when you add more products to your routine.

You don't need to use all of these products, but by reading this guide you now have a much clearer idea of what you might need. So, when you decide to add something to your routine, refer to this sequence to know where it goes.

Here is the **eight-step skincare routine** you should follow twice a day, in the morning and the evening, after you shower/bathe.

01	Cleanser
02	Toner
03	Serum
04	Eye Cream
05	Spot Treatment
06	Moisturizer
07	Face Oil
08	Sunscreen (only in the morning)

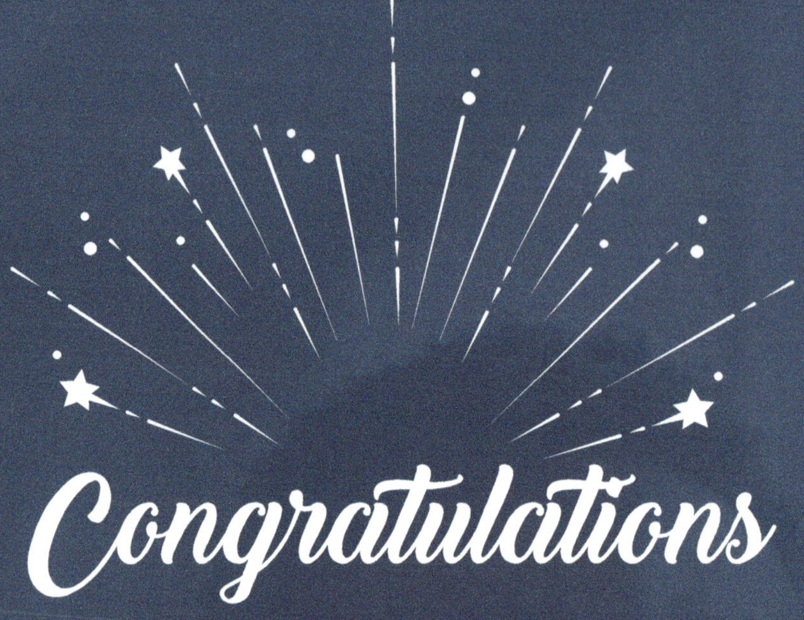

Congratulations

Now you know all you need to get started on your journey to better skin.

Sounds like a lot? It can be overwhelming, but we hope we made this system simple enough that you won't find it difficult to get started.

REMEMBER:

few things can make you confident like having great skin, especially if you have struggled with skin issues in the past or are struggling right now.

There's nothing like looking in the mirror and seeing beautiful, glowing, young-looking skin! And now, that's firmly in your grasp.

Use the coupon code
"WELCOME5"
Avail **5% DISCOUNT** on your first order!

VIVALUI.COM

vivalui
The Skincare Brand for the *Modern Man*

This guide was brought to you by the **VivaLui team**.

But who are we?

Above all, we are people who **care about men's grooming**. We know what modern, busy men want, and we create great skincare products designed and formulated around that.

We are also the same team behind the top beard care brand Castlebeard.

Here at VivaLui, we focus on skincare products that:

Are **formulated specifically for men**, uniting the latest scientific evidence to natural ingredients. We are constantly innovating our formulas to bring maximum results.

Are formulated to be **as delicate and gentle as possible**, to suit every skin type. We don't like aggressive ingredients that do more damage than they help.

Are easy and quick to use to **maximize efficiency and time management**. We don't like products that complicate your life, and that's just what busy men need.

We hope you enjoyed this guide! By implementing the tips in this system, you can expect visible improvements in your skin in just a few weeks. All you need to do is be consistent. Remember: by improving your skin, you're improving your overall health too.

Visit our website **vivalui.com** now to read the latest about our skincare solutions designed for men. Use the **coupon code WELCOME5** at checkout for a **5% discount** on your first order!

All our products come with a 60 days guarantee.

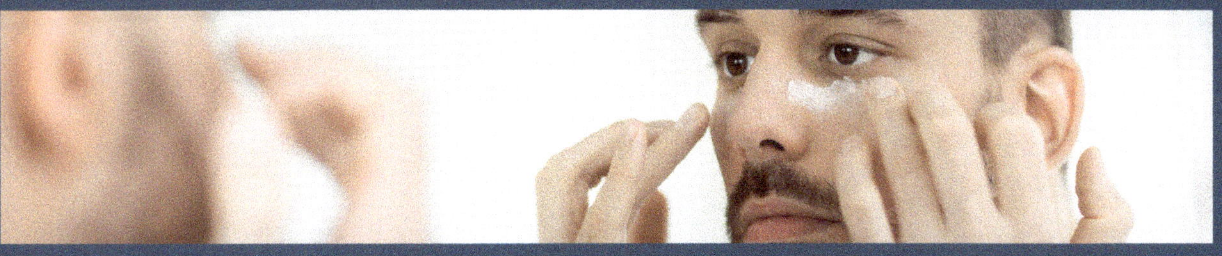